Vertigo Victories

Conquering Meniere's Disease for a Life of Balance and Clarity

by

Elizabeth Owens

Copyright

CONTENTS

Introduction

Meniere's disease is a chronic disorder of the inner ear that can have a significant impact on an individual's quality of life. Named after the French physician Prosper Meniere who first described it in 1861, this condition is characterized by recurring episodes of vertigo, fluctuating hearing loss, tinnitus (ringing or buzzing in the ear), and a sensation of fullness or pressure in the affected ear.

Symptoms and Diagnosis

The hallmark symptoms of Meniere's disease can vary in intensity and duration from person to person. Episodes of vertigo can be particularly debilitating, causing a sensation of spinning or whirling that can last for minutes to hours. These episodes are often accompanied by nausea, vomiting, and a feeling of unsteadiness or imbalance.

Hearing loss associated with Meniere's disease is typically sensorineural, affecting the ability to hear sounds clearly, especially low-frequency sounds. Tinnitus is also common and can manifest as ringing, buzzing, or roaring noises in the ear. The sensation of fullness or pressure in the ear may precede or accompany vertigo attacks.

Diagnosing Meniere's disease can be challenging as there is no specific test for it. Instead, healthcare providers rely on a combination of medical history, physical examination, and a series of tests, including hearing tests (audiometry), balance tests (electronystagmography or ENG), and imaging studies (MRI or CT scans) to rule out other possible causes of symptoms.

Causes and Triggers

The exact cause of Meniere's disease is not fully understood, but it is believed to be related to an abnormal buildup of fluid (endolymph) in the inner ear. This fluid imbalance can disrupt the normal function of the inner ear, leading to the characteristic symptoms of the condition. Several factors may contribute to this fluid buildup, including:

- Abnormalities in the fluid-regulating systems of the inner ear
- Allergies
- Autoimmune response
- Genetics
- Viral infections

Triggers for Meniere's disease episodes can vary from person to person but may include stress, changes in barometric pressure, certain foods (especially those high in salt), caffeine, alcohol, and fatigue.

Impact on Daily Life

Meniere's disease can have a significant impact on various aspects of daily life. The unpredictable nature of vertigo attacks can make it challenging to engage in activities that require balance or concentration. Hearing loss and tinnitus can affect communication, social interactions, and work performance. The emotional toll of living with a chronic condition, coupled with the uncertainty of when symptoms may occur, can lead to anxiety, depression, and a sense of isolation.

In this guidebook, we will explore strategies for managing Meniere's disease, focusing on dietary modifications, physical therapy, and stress management techniques that can help individuals cope with the symptoms and improve their overall well-being. By understanding the nature of Meniere's disease and learning how to effectively manage its symptoms, individuals can take control of their health and lead fulfilling lives despite the challenges posed by this condition.

Chapter 1: Understanding

Meniere's Disease

Meniere's disease is a chronic disorder of the inner ear that can cause a range of symptoms, including vertigo (a spinning sensation), fluctuating hearing loss, tinnitus (ringing in the ears), and a feeling of fullness or pressure in the affected ear. These symptoms can vary in intensity and duration, often occurring in episodes that can last from minutes to hours. While the exact cause of Meniere's disease is not fully understood, it is believed to be related to fluid buildup in the inner ear, leading to changes in hearing and balance.

Symptoms of Meniere's Disease

- Vertigo: A hallmark symptom of Meniere's disease, vertigo is a sensation of spinning or dizziness that can be severe and disabling. It is often accompanied by nausea, vomiting, and a loss of balance.

- Fluctuating Hearing Loss: People with Meniere's disease may experience episodes of hearing loss that come and go, typically affecting one ear. This hearing loss is often low-frequency at first but can progress to involve higher frequencies over time.

- Tinnitus: Many individuals with Meniere's disease experience tinnitus, which is the perception of ringing, buzzing, or other noises in the ear. This symptom can be constant or intermittent and may vary in intensity.

- Ear Fullness: A feeling of fullness or pressure in the affected ear is common in Meniere's disease, often preceding or accompanying vertigo episodes.

Diagnosis of Meniere's Disease

Diagnosing Meniere's disease can be challenging due to the variability of symptoms and the absence of specific diagnostic tests. Healthcare providers typically rely on a combination of medical history, symptoms, and various tests to make a diagnosis. These may include:

- Audiometric Testing: A hearing test to assess the extent and nature of hearing loss.

- Vestibular Testing: Tests that evaluate balance and inner ear function, such as videonystagmography (VNG) or electronystagmography (ENG).
- Imaging Studies: In some cases, imaging studies like magnetic resonance imaging (MRI) may be used to rule out other potential causes of symptoms.

It is essential for individuals experiencing symptoms of Meniere's disease to seek evaluation by a healthcare professional specializing in ear disorders. Early diagnosis and treatment can help manage symptoms and improve quality of life for those living with this condition.

Causes and Triggers

The exact cause of Meniere's disease remains unclear, but it is believed to result from a combination of factors that affect the fluid balance in the inner ear. The inner ear contains structures responsible for both hearing and balance, including the cochlea (responsible for hearing) and the vestibular system (responsible for balance). Changes in the fluid volume or composition within these structures can lead to the characteristic symptoms of Meniere's disease.

Several theories exist regarding the underlying causes of Meniere's disease, including:

1. Endolymphatic Hydrops: This is a condition where there is an excessive accumulation of fluid (endolymph) within the inner ear. It is considered one of the primary contributors to the development of Meniere's disease. The reasons for the abnormal accumulation of endolymph are not fully understood, but it is believed to be related to dysfunction in the regulation or absorption of this fluid.

2. Vascular Disorders: Some researchers believe that changes in the blood vessels supplying the inner ear could contribute to the development of Meniere's disease. This theory suggests that alterations in blood flow to the inner ear could lead to changes in fluid dynamics, contributing to symptoms.

3. Autoimmune Factors: There is evidence to suggest that autoimmune mechanisms may play a role in some cases of Meniere's disease. In autoimmune disorders, the body's immune system mistakenly attacks its own tissues, leading to inflammation and tissue damage. In the case of Meniere's disease,

autoimmune factors could potentially affect the inner ear, leading to symptoms.

Triggers for Meniere's Disease

While the exact causes of Meniere's disease are not fully understood, certain triggers or factors can exacerbate symptoms or contribute to the onset of episodes. These triggers can vary from person to person, but some common ones include:

1. Dietary Factors: Excessive salt intake is a well-known trigger for Meniere's disease, as it can lead to fluid retention and changes in inner ear fluid balance. Caffeine and alcohol are also known to affect some individuals with Meniere's disease, potentially triggering symptoms.

2. Stress and Anxiety: Emotional stress and anxiety can exacerbate symptoms of Meniere's disease, particularly vertigo. Stress management techniques can be an important part of managing the condition.

3. Changes in Atmospheric Pressure: Some individuals with Meniere's disease may be sensitive to changes in

atmospheric pressure, such as those experienced during air travel or changes in weather patterns.

4. Certain Medications: Some medications can affect the inner ear or have side effects that worsen symptoms of Meniere's disease. It is essential to discuss medication use with a healthcare provider to ensure that any potential triggers are identified and managed.

Impact on Daily Life

Meniere's disease can have a profound impact on an individual's daily life due to its unpredictable nature and the range of symptoms it presents. The hallmark symptoms of Meniere's—vertigo, hearing loss, tinnitus, and ear fullness—can significantly disrupt various aspects of daily living, including work, social interactions, and leisure activities.

1. Work and Productivity:
   - Vertigo attacks can be sudden and severe, making it challenging to maintain regular work schedules.
   - The fluctuating nature of symptoms may lead to unpredictable absences from work, affecting productivity and performance.

- Concentration and focus may be compromised during vertigo episodes, impacting the ability to perform tasks that require attention to detail.

2. Social Interactions:
   - Socializing may become more challenging due to the fear of experiencing vertigo attacks in public settings.
   - Hearing loss and tinnitus can affect communication, making it difficult to follow conversations in noisy environments.
   - The need for dietary restrictions (such as avoiding salty foods) may limit dining out with friends or family.

3. Emotional Well-being:
   - Coping with the unpredictable nature of Meniere's disease can lead to feelings of anxiety and stress.
   - The impact of symptoms on daily life may lead to feelings of isolation and frustration.
   - Managing the emotional toll of Meniere's, along with its physical symptoms, is essential for overall well-being.

4. Leisure Activities:
   - Hobbies and recreational activities may be limited due to concerns about triggering vertigo attacks.

- Activities that require good balance, such as certain sports or outdoor activities, may need to be adapted or avoided.
- Planning leisure activities around symptom patterns and triggers becomes necessary to minimize the impact of Meniere's on enjoyment and participation.

Chapter 2. Dietary Modifications for Meniere's Disease

Role of Diet in Managing Symptoms

Diet plays a crucial role in managing Meniere's disease by influencing the fluid balance in the inner ear. Excessive fluid buildup in the inner ear is believed to contribute to the development of symptoms such as vertigo, tinnitus, and ear fullness. By making strategic dietary modifications, individuals with Meniere's can potentially reduce the frequency and severity of their symptoms and improve their overall quality of life.

1. Sodium and Fluid Balance:

- High sodium intake can lead to fluid retention in the body, including the inner ear, exacerbating symptoms of Meniere's disease.
- A low-sodium diet is commonly recommended for individuals with Meniere's to help regulate fluid balance and reduce the pressure in the inner ear.
- By reducing sodium intake, individuals may experience a decrease in the severity and frequency of vertigo attacks and other symptoms associated with Meniere's.

2. Trigger Foods:
- Certain foods and beverages, such as those high in sodium, caffeine, or alcohol, may act as triggers for Meniere's symptoms in some individuals.
- Identifying and avoiding these trigger foods can help manage symptoms and improve overall well-being.
- Keeping a food diary to track dietary intake and symptom patterns can be beneficial in identifying specific triggers.

3. Hydration:
- Adequate hydration is essential for overall health, including maintaining proper fluid balance in the body.

- While it may seem counterintuitive, staying well-hydrated can actually help prevent fluid retention in the inner ear by promoting proper fluid circulation.
- Balancing hydration with sodium intake is important, as excessive fluid intake without proper sodium regulation can also impact symptoms.

Low-Sodium Diet: Benefits and Practical Tips

A low-sodium diet is a cornerstone of dietary management for Meniere's disease, as it can help reduce fluid retention in the inner ear, potentially alleviating symptoms such as vertigo and ear fullness. By understanding the benefits of a low-sodium diet and implementing practical tips for reducing sodium intake, individuals with Meniere's can take an active role in managing their condition.

Benefits of a Low-Sodium Diet:
1. Fluid Balance: Sodium plays a key role in regulating fluid balance in the body, including the inner ear. By reducing sodium intake, individuals can help maintain a more stable fluid balance, potentially reducing the severity and frequency of vertigo attacks.

2. Blood Pressure Management: A low-sodium diet is also beneficial for managing blood pressure, which is important for overall cardiovascular health. Since hypertension (high blood pressure) can exacerbate Meniere's symptoms, maintaining healthy blood pressure levels is crucial.

3. Minimizing Symptom Triggers: Many individuals with Meniere's find that certain foods high in sodium can trigger or worsen their symptoms. By identifying and avoiding these trigger foods, individuals can better control their symptoms and improve their quality of life.

Practical Tips for a Low-Sodium Diet:

1. Read Food Labels: Pay close attention to the sodium content listed on food labels. Choose products labeled "low sodium" or "sodium-free" whenever possible.

2. Cook at Home: Prepare meals at home using fresh, whole ingredients, which tend to be lower in sodium than processed or pre-packaged foods.

3. Use Herbs and Spices: Instead of salt, flavor foods with herbs, spices, and citrus juices to enhance taste without adding sodium.

4. Be Mindful When Dining Out: When eating out, ask for sauces and dressings on the side to control sodium intake. Choose restaurants that offer low-sodium options or are willing to accommodate dietary restrictions.

5. Limit Processed Foods: Processed foods, such as canned soups, deli meats, and packaged snacks, are often high in sodium. Limiting these foods can significantly reduce sodium intake.

6. Monitor Fluid Intake: In addition to sodium, monitoring fluid intake, especially caffeine and alcohol, can help manage symptoms related to fluid balance.

Identifying Trigger Foods

One key aspect of managing Meniere's disease through dietary modifications is identifying and avoiding trigger foods that may exacerbate symptoms. While trigger foods can vary from person to person, there are some common culprits that individuals with

Meniere's may want to be cautious about including in their diets.

1. High-Sodium Foods:
   - Foods high in sodium can contribute to fluid retention in the body, including the inner ear, which can worsen symptoms of Meniere's disease.
   - Common sources of high sodium include processed foods (e.g., canned soups, deli meats, snacks), fast food, and restaurant meals.
   - Reading food labels and choosing low-sodium or sodium-free alternatives can help reduce sodium intake.

2. Caffeine and Alcohol:
   - Both caffeine and alcohol are known to affect fluid balance in the body and can potentially trigger or worsen vertigo and other symptoms of Meniere's.
   - Limiting or avoiding caffeinated beverages (e.g., coffee, tea, energy drinks) and alcoholic beverages may help some individuals manage their symptoms better.

3. Certain Food Additives:
   - Some food additives, such as monosodium glutamate (MSG), artificial sweeteners (e.g.,

aspartame), and nitrates/nitrites (found in processed meats), have been reported to trigger symptoms in some people with Meniere's.
  - Reading ingredient labels and choosing foods without these additives can be beneficial for those sensitive to them.

4. Other Potential Triggers:
  - While individual sensitivities can vary widely, some people with Meniere's report sensitivity to specific foods like chocolate, aged cheeses, and certain fruits.
  - Keeping a food diary to track symptoms in relation to food intake can help identify patterns and pinpoint potential trigger foods.

5. Fluid Intake:
  - Maintaining adequate hydration is important for overall health, but individuals with Meniere's may need to be mindful of their fluid intake, especially if they are prone to fluid retention.
  - Drinking plenty of water and choosing hydrating foods like fruits and vegetables can help maintain proper fluid balance without overloading the system.

Importance of Hydration

Hydration plays a crucial role in managing Meniere's disease, as maintaining proper fluid balance can help alleviate symptoms and support overall health. Adequate hydration is essential for the body's various functions, including regulating blood pressure and maintaining the balance of fluids in the inner ear.

1. Fluid Balance in the Inner Ear:
   - The inner ear relies on a delicate balance of fluids to function properly.
   - Changes in fluid balance can affect the pressure in the inner ear, potentially triggering symptoms like vertigo and ear fullness.

2. Effects of Dehydration:
   - Dehydration can exacerbate symptoms of Meniere's disease, as it may lead to changes in fluid volume and pressure within the inner ear.
   - Symptoms such as dizziness, lightheadedness, and fatigue can be more pronounced when the body is not adequately hydrated.

3. Importance of Proper Hydration:
   - Maintaining proper hydration levels can help stabilize fluid pressure in the inner ear, potentially reducing the frequency and severity of vertigo attacks.
   - Adequate hydration is also essential for overall health and well-being, supporting the body's various physiological processes.

4. Tips for Staying Hydrated:
   - Drink plenty of water throughout the day, aiming for at least eight 8-ounce glasses per day.
   - Limit the consumption of dehydrating beverages such as caffeinated and alcoholic drinks.
   - Monitor urine color as a simple indicator of hydration status—pale yellow urine indicates adequate hydration, while dark yellow urine may indicate dehydration.

5. Hydration and Dietary Modifications:
   - Hydration is closely linked to dietary modifications for Meniere's disease, particularly in the context of managing sodium intake.
   - Balancing fluid intake with sodium restriction is important for maintaining overall fluid balance and minimizing symptoms.

Chapter 3. Meal Planning for

Meniere's

Sample Menus for Low-Sodium Meals (<2000mg daily)

Day 1
Breakfast:
- Oatmeal (1/2 cup dry): 150 calories, 27g carbs, 4g protein, 3g fat, 0mg sodium
- Banana (1 medium): 105 calories, 27g carbs, 1g protein, 0g fat, 1mg sodium

- Total: 255 calories, 54g carbs, 5g protein, 3g fat, 1mg sodium

Lunch:
- Turkey Sandwich (2 slices whole wheat bread, 2 oz turkey breast, lettuce, tomato): 300 calories, 30g carbs, 22g protein, 10g fat, 600mg sodium (approx.)

- Apple (1 medium): 95 calories, 25g carbs, 0g protein, 0g fat, 2mg sodium

- Total: 395 calories, 55g carbs, 22g protein, 10g fat, 602mg sodium (approx.)

Dinner:
- Grilled Chicken Breast (4 oz): 185 calories, 0g carbs, 35g protein, 4g fat, 75mg sodium (approx.)
- Quinoa (1/2 cup cooked): 111 calories, 19g carbs, 4g protein, 2g fat, 7mg sodium
- Steamed Broccoli (1 cup): 55 calories, 11g carbs, 4g protein, 1g fat, 30mg sodium (approx.)

- Total: 351 calories, 30g carbs, 43g protein, 7g fat, 112mg sodium (approx.)

Snack:
- Greek Yogurt (6 oz): 100 calories, 9g carbs, 17g protein, 0g fat, 60mg sodium (approx.)

- Total: 100 calories, 9g carbs, 17g protein, 0g fat, 60mg sodium (approx.)

Day 2
Breakfast:

- Scrambled Eggs (2 large eggs): 140 calories, 2g carbs, 12g protein, 9g fat, 140mg sodium (approx.)
- Whole Wheat Toast (2 slices): 160 calories, 28g carbs, 6g protein, 2g fat, 240mg sodium (approx.)

- Total: 300 calories, 30g carbs, 18g protein, 11g fat, 380mg sodium (approx.)

Lunch:
- Tuna Salad (3 oz canned tuna, mixed greens, cherry tomatoes, cucumber, olive oil, lemon juice): 200 calories, 5g carbs, 20g protein, 10g fat, 350mg sodium (approx.)

- Whole Grain Crackers (6 crackers): 120 calories, 20g carbs, 3g protein, 3g fat, 200mg sodium (approx.)

- Total: 320 calories, 25g carbs, 23g protein, 13g fat, 550mg sodium (approx.)

Dinner:
- Baked Salmon (4 oz): 220 calories, 0g carbs, 23g protein, 13g fat, 70mg sodium (approx.)
- Brown Rice (1/2 cup cooked): 108 calories, 22g carbs, 2g protein, 1g fat, 2mg sodium

- Steamed Asparagus (1/2 cup): 20 calories, 4g carbs, 2g protein, 0g fat, 0mg sodium

- Total: 348 calories, 26g carbs, 27g protein, 14g fat, 72mg sodium (approx.)

Snack:
- Carrot Sticks (1 cup): 50 calories, 12g carbs, 1g protein, 0g fat, 70mg sodium (approx.)
- Hummus (2 tbsp): 70 calories, 6g carbs, 2g protein, 4g fat, 140mg sodium (approx.)

- Total: 120 calories, 18g carbs, 3g protein, 4g fat, 210mg sodium (approx.)

Day 3
Breakfast:
- Greek Yogurt (6 oz): 100 calories, 9g carbs, 17g protein, 0g fat, 60mg sodium (approx.)
- Mixed Berries (1/2 cup): 40 calories, 10g carbs, 1g protein, 0g fat, 0mg sodium

- Total: 140 calories, 19g carbs, 18g protein, 0g fat, 60mg sodium (approx.)

Lunch:

- Turkey and Avocado Wrap (2 slices turkey, 1/4 avocado, lettuce, tomato, whole wheat wrap): 300 calories, 30g carbs, 22g protein, 10g fat, 600mg sodium (approx.)
- Orange (1 medium): 62 calories, 15g carbs, 1g protein, 0g fat, 0mg sodium

- Total: 362 calories, 45g carbs, 23g protein, 10g fat, 600mg sodium (approx.)

Dinner:
- Grilled Chicken Caesar Salad (4 oz grilled chicken breast, romaine lettuce, cherry tomatoes, Caesar dressing): 350 calories, 8g carbs, 40g protein, 18g fat, 700mg sodium (approx.)
- Whole Grain Breadstick: 100 calories, 20g carbs, 3g protein, 1g fat, 200mg sodium (approx.)

- Total: 450 calories, 28g carbs, 43g protein, 19g fat, 900mg sodium (approx.)

Snack:
- Almonds (1/4 cup): 206 calories, 8g carbs, 8g protein, 18g fat, 0mg sodium

- Total: 206 calories, 8g carbs, 8g protein, 18g fat, 0mg sodium

Day 4
Breakfast:
- Whole Grain Pancakes (2 pancakes): 200 calories, 40g carbs, 6g protein, 2g fat, 400mg sodium (approx.)
- Fresh Strawberries (1/2 cup): 24 calories, 6g carbs, 0g protein, 0g fat, 1mg sodium

- Total: 224 calories, 46g carbs, 6g protein, 2g fat, 401mg sodium (approx.)

Lunch:
- Veggie Burger (1 patty): 150 calories, 15g carbs, 10g protein, 5g fat, 300mg sodium (approx.)
- Whole Wheat Bun: 120 calories, 24g carbs, 5g protein, 1g fat, 230mg sodium (approx.)

- Total: 270 calories, 39g carbs, 15g protein, 6g fat, 530mg sodium (approx.)

Dinner:
- Shrimp Stir-Fry (4 oz shrimp, mixed vegetables, soy sauce): 200 calories, 10g carbs, 25g protein, 6g fat, 700mg sodium (approx.)

- Brown Rice (1/2 cup cooked): 108 calories, 22g carbs, 2g protein, 1g fat, 2mg sodium

- Total: 308 calories, 32g carbs, 27g protein, 7g fat, 702mg sodium (approx.)

Snack:
- Cottage Cheese (1/2 cup): 110 calories, 6g carbs, 14g protein, 4g fat, 400mg sodium (approx.)

- Total: 110 calories, 6g carbs, 14g protein, 4g fat, 400mg sodium (approx.)

Day 5
Breakfast:
- Greek Yogurt (6 oz): 100 calories, 9g carbs, 17g protein, 0g fat, 60mg sodium (approx.)
- Mixed Berries (1/2 cup): 40 calories, 10g carbs, 1g protein, 0g fat, 0mg sodium

- Total: 140 calories, 19g carbs, 18g protein, 0g fat, 60mg sodium (approx.)

Lunch:
- Turkey and Swiss Cheese Wrap (2 slices turkey, 1 slice Swiss cheese, lettuce, tomato, whole wheat wrap): 300

calories, 30g carbs, 23g protein, 10g fat, 550mg sodium (approx.)
- Carrot Sticks (1 cup): 50 calories, 12g carbs, 1g protein, 0g fat, 70mg sodium (approx.)

- Total: 350 calories, 42g carbs, 24g protein, 10g fat, 620mg sodium (approx.)

Dinner:
- Grilled Salmon (4 oz): 220 calories, 0g carbs, 23g protein, 13g fat, 70mg sodium (approx.)
- Quinoa (1/2 cup cooked): 111 calories, 19g carbs, 4g protein, 2g fat, 7mg sodium
- Steamed Spinach (1/2 cup): 21 calories, 3g carbs, 3g protein, 0g fat, 50mg sodium (approx.)

- Total: 352 calories, 22g carbs, 30g protein, 15g fat, 127mg sodium (approx.)

Snack:
- Cottage Cheese (1/2 cup): 110 calories, 6g carbs, 14g protein, 4g fat, 400mg sodium (approx.)

- Total: 110 calories, 6g carbs, 14g protein, 4g fat, 400mg sodium (approx.)

Day 6
Breakfast:
- Whole Grain Toast with Almond Butter (2 slices toast, 2 tbsp almond butter): 300 calories, 30g carbs, 10g protein, 16g fat, 200mg sodium (approx.)
- Sliced Pear (1 medium): 100 calories, 25g carbs, 1g protein, 0g fat, 0mg sodium

- Total: 400 calories, 55g carbs, 11g protein, 16g fat, 200mg sodium (approx.)

Lunch:
- Grilled Chicken Salad (4 oz grilled chicken breast, mixed greens, cherry tomatoes, cucumber, balsamic vinaigrette): 250 calories, 8g carbs, 35g protein, 8g fat, 400mg sodium (approx.)
- Whole Grain Crackers (6 crackers): 120 calories, 20g carbs, 3g protein, 3g fat, 200mg sodium (approx.)

- Total: 370 calories, 28g carbs, 38g protein, 11g fat, 600mg sodium (approx.)

Dinner:
- Baked Cod (4 oz): 150 calories, 0g carbs, 30g protein, 2g fat, 75mg sodium (approx.)

- Quinoa (1/2 cup cooked): 111 calories, 19g carbs, 4g protein, 2g fat, 7mg sodium
- Steamed Broccoli (1/2 cup): 55 calories, 11g carbs, 4g protein, 1g fat, 30mg sodium (approx.)

- Total: 316 calories, 30g carbs, 38g protein, 5g fat, 112mg sodium (approx.)

Snack:
- Greek Yogurt with Honey (6 oz): 150 calories, 20g carbs, 11g protein, 0g fat, 70mg sodium (approx.)

- Total: 150 calories, 20g carbs, 11g protein, 0g fat, 70mg sodium (approx.)

Day 7
Breakfast:
- Scrambled Eggs with Spinach (2 large eggs, 1/2 cup spinach): 160 calories, 2g carbs, 13g protein, 11g fat, 140mg sodium (approx.)
- Whole Wheat English Muffin: 120 calories, 24g carbs, 5g protein, 1g fat, 200mg sodium (approx.)

- Total: 280 calories, 26g carbs, 18g protein, 12g fat, 340mg sodium (approx.)

Lunch:
- Turkey and Hummus Wrap (2 slices turkey, 2 tbsp hummus, lettuce, tomato, whole wheat wrap): 300 calories, 30g carbs, 22g protein, 10g fat, 600mg sodium (approx.)
- Orange (1 medium): 62 calories, 15g carbs, 1g protein, 0g fat, 0mg sodium

- Total: 362 calories, 45g carbs, 23g protein, 10g fat, 600mg sodium (approx.)

Dinner:
- Grilled Steak (4 oz): 250 calories, 0g carbs, 28g protein, 15g fat, 60mg sodium (approx.)
- Roasted Sweet Potatoes (1/2 cup): 90 calories, 20g carbs, 1g protein, 0g fat, 70mg sodium (approx.)
- Steamed Green Beans (1/2 cup): 20 calories, 4g carbs, 1g protein, 0g fat, 1mg sodium

- Total: 360 calories, 24g carbs, 30g protein, 15g fat, 131mg sodium (approx.)

Snack:
- Apple with Almond Butter (1 medium apple, 2 tbsp almond butter): 250 calories, 25g carbs, 4g protein, 16g fat, 0mg sodium

- Total: 250 calories, 25g carbs, 4g protein, 16g fat, 0mg sodium

Day 8
Breakfast:
- Whole Grain Pancakes with Berries (2 pancakes, 1/2 cup mixed berries): 260 calories, 52g carbs, 6g protein, 2g fat, 490mg sodium (approx.)

- Total: 260 calories, 52g carbs, 6g protein, 2g fat, 490mg sodium (approx.)

Lunch:
- Grilled Chicken Caesar Salad (4 oz grilled chicken breast, romaine lettuce, cherry tomatoes, Caesar dressing): 350 calories, 8g carbs, 40g protein, 18g fat, 700mg sodium (approx.)
- Whole Grain Breadstick: 100 calories, 20g carbs, 3g protein, 1g fat, 200mg sodium (approx.)

- Total: 450 calories, 28g carbs, 43g protein, 19g fat, 900mg sodium (approx.)

Dinner:

- Baked Tilapia (4 oz): 120 calories, 0g carbs, 23g protein, 3g fat, 55mg sodium (approx.)
- Quinoa (1/2 cup cooked): 111 calories, 19g carbs, 4g protein, 2g fat, 7mg sodium
- Steamed Broccoli (1/2 cup): 55 calories, 11g carbs, 4g protein, 1g fat, 30mg sodium (approx.)

- Total: 286 calories, 30g carbs, 31g protein, 6g fat, 92mg sodium (approx.)

Snack:
- Greek Yogurt with Honey (6 oz): 150 calories, 20g carbs, 11g protein, 0g fat, 70mg sodium (approx.)

- Total: 150 calories, 20g carbs, 11g protein, 0g fat, 70mg sodium (approx.)

Day 9
Breakfast:
- Scrambled Eggs with Spinach (2 large eggs, 1/2 cup spinach): 160 calories, 2g carbs, 13g protein, 11g fat, 140mg sodium (approx.)
- Whole Wheat English Muffin: 120 calories, 24g carbs, 5g protein, 1g fat, 200mg sodium (approx.)

- Total: 280 calories, 26g carbs, 18g protein, 12g fat, 340mg sodium (approx.)

Lunch:
- Turkey and Hummus Wrap (2 slices turkey, 2 tbsp hummus, lettuce, tomato, whole wheat wrap): 300 calories, 30g carbs, 22g protein, 10g fat, 600mg sodium (approx.)
- Orange (1 medium): 62 calories, 15g carbs, 1g protein, 0g fat, 0mg sodium

- Total: 362 calories, 45g carbs, 23g protein, 10g fat, 600mg sodium (approx.)

Dinner:
- Grilled Steak (4 oz): 250 calories, 0g carbs, 28g protein, 15g fat, 60mg sodium (approx.)
- Roasted Sweet Potatoes (1/2 cup): 90 calories, 20g carbs, 1g protein, 0g fat, 70mg sodium (approx.)
- Steamed Green Beans (1/2 cup): 20 calories, 4g carbs, 1g protein, 0g fat, 1mg sodium

- Total: 360 calories, 24g carbs, 30g protein, 15g fat, 131mg sodium (approx.)

Snack:

- Apple with Almond Butter (1 medium apple, 2 tbsp almond butter): 250 calories, 25g carbs, 4g protein, 16g fat, 0mg sodium

- Total: 250 calories, 25g carbs, 4g protein, 16g fat, 0mg sodium

Day 10
Breakfast:
- Greek Yogurt (6 oz): 100 calories, 9g carbs, 17g protein, 0g fat, 60mg sodium (approx.)
- Mixed Berries (1/2 cup): 40 calories, 10g carbs, 1g protein, 0g fat, 0mg sodium

- Total: 140 calories, 19g carbs, 18g protein, 0g fat, 60mg sodium (approx.)

Lunch:
- Turkey and Swiss Cheese Wrap (2 slices turkey, 1 slice Swiss cheese, lettuce, tomato, whole wheat wrap): 300 calories, 30g carbs, 23g protein, 10g fat, 550mg sodium (approx.)
- Carrot Sticks (1 cup): 50 calories, 12g carbs, 1g protein, 0g fat, 70mg sodium (approx.)

- Total: 350 calories, 42g carbs, 24g protein, 10g fat, 620mg sodium (approx.)

Dinner:
- Grilled Salmon (4 oz): 220 calories, 0g carbs, 23g protein, 13g fat, 70mg sodium (approx.)
- Quinoa (1/2 cup cooked): 111 calories, 19g carbs, 4g protein, 2g fat, 7mg sodium
- Steamed Spinach (1/2 cup): 21 calories, 3g carbs, 3g protein, 0g fat, 50mg sodium (approx.)

- Total: 352 calories, 22g carbs, 30g protein, 15g fat, 127mg sodium (approx.)

Snack:
- Cottage Cheese (1/2 cup): 110 calories, 6g carbs, 14g protein, 4g fat, 400mg sodium (approx.)

- Total: 110 calories, 6g carbs, 14g protein, 4g fat, 400mg sodium (approx.)

Day 11
Breakfast:
- Whole Grain Toast with Almond Butter (2 slices toast, 2 tbsp almond butter): 300 calories, 30g carbs, 10g protein, 16g fat, 200mg sodium (approx.)

- Sliced Pear (1 medium): 100 calories, 25g carbs, 1g protein, 0g fat, 0mg sodium

- Total: 400 calories, 55g carbs, 11g protein, 16g fat, 200mg sodium (approx.)

Lunch:
- Grilled Chicken Salad (4 oz grilled chicken breast, mixed greens, cherry tomatoes, cucumber, balsamic vinaigrette): 250 calories, 8g carbs, 35g protein, 8g fat, 400mg sodium (approx.)
- Whole Grain Crackers (6 crackers): 120 calories, 20g carbs, 3g protein, 3g fat, 200mg sodium (approx.)

- Total: 370 calories, 28g carbs, 38g protein, 11g fat, 600mg sodium (approx.)

Dinner:
- Baked Cod (4 oz): 120 calories, 0g carbs, 23g protein, 3g fat, 55mg sodium (approx.)
- Quinoa (1/2 cup cooked): 111 calories, 19g carbs, 4g protein, 2g fat, 7mg sodium
- Steamed Broccoli (1/2 cup): 55 calories, 11g carbs, 4g protein, 1g fat, 30mg sodium (approx.)

- Total: 286 calories, 30g carbs, 31g protein, 6g fat, 92mg sodium (approx.)

Snack:
- Greek Yogurt with Honey (6 oz): 150 calories, 20g carbs, 11g protein, 0g fat, 70mg sodium (approx.)

- Total: 150 calories, 20g carbs, 11g protein, 0g fat, 70mg sodium (approx.)

Day 12
Breakfast:
- Scrambled Eggs with Spinach (2 large eggs, 1/2 cup spinach): 160 calories, 2g carbs, 13g protein, 11g fat, 140mg sodium (approx.)
- Whole Wheat English Muffin: 120 calories, 24g carbs, 5g protein, 1g fat, 200mg sodium (approx.)

- Total: 280 calories, 26g carbs, 18g protein, 12g fat, 340mg sodium (approx.)

Lunch:
- Turkey and Hummus Wrap (2 slices turkey, 2 tbsp hummus, lettuce, tomato, whole wheat wrap): 300 calories, 30g carbs, 22g protein, 10g fat, 600mg sodium (approx.)

- Orange (1 medium): 62 calories, 15g carbs, 1g protein, 0g fat, 0mg sodium

- Total: 362 calories, 45g carbs, 23g protein, 10g fat, 600mg sodium (approx.)

Dinner:
- Grilled Steak (4 oz): 250 calories, 0g carbs, 28g protein, 15g fat, 60mg sodium (approx.)
- Roasted Sweet Potatoes (1/2 cup): 90 calories, 20g carbs, 1g protein, 0g fat, 70mg sodium (approx.)
- Steamed Green Beans (1/2 cup): 20 calories, 4g carbs, 1g protein, 0g fat, 1mg sodium

- Total: 360 calories, 24g carbs, 30g protein, 15g fat, 131mg sodium (approx.)

Snack:
- Apple with Almond Butter (1 medium apple, 2 tbsp almond butter): 250 calories, 25g carbs, 4g protein, 16g fat, 0mg sodium

- Total: 250 calories, 25g carbs, 4g protein, 16g fat, 0mg sodium

Day 13

Breakfast:
- Whole Grain Pancakes with Berries (2 pancakes, 1/2 cup mixed berries): 260 calories, 52g carbs, 6g protein, 2g fat, 490mg sodium (approx.)

- Total: 260 calories, 52g carbs, 6g protein, 2g fat, 490mg sodium (approx.)

Lunch:
- Grilled Chicken Caesar Salad (4 oz grilled chicken breast, romaine lettuce, cherry tomatoes, Caesar dressing): 350 calories, 8g carbs, 40g protein, 18g fat, 700mg sodium (approx.)
- Whole Grain Breadstick: 100 calories, 20g carbs, 3g protein, 1g fat, 200mg sodium (approx.)

- Total: 450 calories, 28g carbs, 43g protein, 19g fat, 900mg sodium (approx.)

Dinner:
- Baked Tilapia (4 oz): 120 calories, 0g carbs, 23g protein, 3g fat, 55mg sodium (approx.)
- Quinoa (1/2 cup cooked): 111 calories, 19g carbs, 4g protein, 2g fat, 7mg sodium
- Steamed Broccoli (1/2 cup): 55 calories, 11g carbs, 4g protein, 1g fat, 30mg sodium (approx.)

- Total: 286 calories, 30g carbs, 31g protein, 6g fat, 92mg sodium (approx.)

Snack:
- Greek Yogurt with Honey (6 oz): 150 calories, 20g carbs, 11g protein, 0g fat, 70mg sodium (approx.)

- Total: 150 calories, 20g carbs, 11g protein, 0g fat, 70mg sodium (approx.)

Day 14
Breakfast:
- Greek Yogurt (6 oz): 100 calories, 9g carbs, 17g protein, 0g fat, 60mg sodium (approx.)
- Mixed Berries (1/2 cup): 40 calories, 10g carbs, 1g protein, 0g fat, 0mg sodium

- Total: 140 calories, 19g carbs, 18g protein, 0g fat, 60mg sodium (approx.)

Lunch:
- Turkey and Swiss Cheese Wrap (2 slices turkey, 1 slice Swiss cheese, lettuce, tomato, whole wheat wrap): 300 calories, 30g carbs, 23g protein, 10g fat, 550mg sodium (approx.)

- Carrot Sticks (1 cup): 50 calories, 12g carbs, 1g protein, 0g fat, 70mg sodium (approx.)

- Total: 350 calories, 42g carbs, 24g protein, 10g fat, 620mg sodium (approx.)

Dinner:
- Grilled Salmon (4 oz): 220 calories, 0g carbs, 23g protein, 13g fat, 70mg sodium (approx.)
- Quinoa (1/2 cup cooked): 111 calories, 19g carbs, 4g protein, 2g fat, 7mg sodium
- Steamed Spinach (1/2 cup): 21 calories, 3g carbs, 3g protein, 0g fat, 50mg sodium (approx.)

- Total: 352 calories, 22g carbs, 30g protein, 15g fat, 127mg sodium (approx.)

Snack:
- Cottage Cheese (1/2 cup): 110 calories, 6g carbs, 14g protein, 4g fat, 400mg sodium (approx.)

- Total: 110 calories, 6g carbs, 14g protein, 4g fat, 400mg sodium (approx.)

Day 15
Breakfast:

- Oatmeal with Almond Milk (1/2 cup oats cooked in 1 cup almond milk): 180 calories, 30g carbs, 6g protein, 4g fat, 80mg sodium (approx.)
- Sliced Banana (1 medium): 105 calories, 27g carbs, 1g protein, 0g fat, 1mg sodium

- Total: 285 calories, 57g carbs, 7g protein, 4g fat, 81mg sodium (approx.)

Lunch:
- Tuna Salad (3 oz canned tuna, mixed greens, cherry tomatoes, cucumber, lemon juice): 150 calories, 3g carbs, 20g protein, 7g fat, 250mg sodium (approx.)
- Whole Grain Crackers (6 crackers): 120 calories, 20g carbs, 3g protein, 3g fat, 200mg sodium (approx.)

- Total: 270 calories, 23g carbs, 23g protein, 10g fat, 450mg sodium (approx.)

Dinner:
- Baked Chicken Breast (4 oz): 187 calories, 0g carbs, 35g protein, 4g fat, 85mg sodium (approx.)
- Quinoa (1/2 cup cooked): 111 calories, 19g carbs, 4g protein, 2g fat, 7mg sodium
- Steamed Asparagus (1/2 cup): 20 calories, 4g carbs, 2g protein, 0g fat, 0mg sodium

- Total: 318 calories, 23g carbs, 41g protein, 6g fat, 92mg sodium (approx.)

Snack:
- Apple Slices with Peanut Butter (1 medium apple, 2 tbsp peanut butter): 250 calories, 26g carbs, 5g protein, 16g fat, 0mg sodium

- Total: 250 calories, 26g carbs, 5g protein, 16g fat, 0mg sodium

Day 16
Breakfast:
- Greek Yogurt with Berries (6 oz Greek yogurt, 1/2 cup mixed berries): 150 calories, 20g carbs, 15g protein, 0g fat, 80mg sodium (approx.)

- Total: 150 calories, 20g carbs, 15g protein, 0g fat, 80mg sodium (approx.)

Lunch:
- Turkey and Avocado Wrap (2 slices turkey, 1/4 avocado, lettuce, tomato, whole wheat wrap): 300 calories, 30g carbs, 23g protein, 12g fat, 550mg sodium (approx.)

- Carrot Sticks (1 cup): 50 calories, 12g carbs, 1g protein, 0g fat, 70mg sodium (approx.)

- Total: 350 calories, 42g carbs, 24g protein, 12g fat, 620mg sodium (approx.)

Dinner:
- Grilled Salmon (4 oz): 220 calories, 0g carbs, 23g protein, 13g fat, 70mg sodium (approx.)
- Brown Rice (1/2 cup cooked): 108 calories, 22g carbs, 2g protein, 1g fat, 2mg sodium
- Steamed Broccoli (1/2 cup): 27 calories, 5g carbs, 2g protein, 0g fat, 30mg sodium (approx.)

- Total: 355 calories, 49g carbs, 27g protein, 14g fat, 102mg sodium (approx.)

Snack:
- Cottage Cheese (1/2 cup): 110 calories, 6g carbs, 14g protein, 4g fat, 400mg sodium (approx.)

- Total: 110 calories, 6g carbs, 14g protein, 4g fat, 400mg sodium (approx.)

Day 17
Breakfast:

- Whole Grain Toast with Almond Butter (2 slices toast, 2 tbsp almond butter): 300 calories, 30g carbs, 10g protein, 16g fat, 200mg sodium (approx.)
- Sliced Pear (1 medium): 100 calories, 25g carbs, 1g protein, 0g fat, 0mg sodium

- Total: 400 calories, 55g carbs, 11g protein, 16g fat, 200mg sodium (approx.)

Lunch:
- Grilled Chicken Salad (4 oz grilled chicken breast, mixed greens, cherry tomatoes, cucumber, balsamic vinaigrette): 250 calories, 8g carbs, 35g protein, 8g fat, 400mg sodium (approx.)
- Whole Grain Crackers (6 crackers): 120 calories, 20g carbs, 3g protein, 3g fat, 200mg sodium (approx.)

- Total: 370 calories, 28g carbs, 38g protein, 11g fat, 600mg sodium (approx.)

Dinner:
- Baked Cod (4 oz): 120 calories, 0g carbs, 23g protein, 3g fat, 55mg sodium (approx.)
- Quinoa (1/2 cup cooked): 111 calories, 19g carbs, 4g protein, 2g fat, 7mg sodium

- Steamed Broccoli (1/2 cup): 55 calories, 11g carbs, 4g protein, 1g fat, 30mg sodium (approx.)

- Total: 286 calories, 30g carbs, 31g protein, 6g fat, 92mg sodium (approx.)

Snack:
- Greek Yogurt with Honey (6 oz): 150 calories, 20g carbs, 11g protein, 0g fat, 70mg sodium (approx.)

- Total: 150 calories, 20g carbs, 11g protein, 0g fat, 70mg sodium (approx.)

Day 18
Breakfast:
- Scrambled Eggs with Spinach (2 large eggs, 1/2 cup spinach): 160 calories, 2g carbs, 13g protein, 11g fat, 140mg sodium (approx.)
- Whole Wheat English Muffin: 120 calories, 24g carbs, 5g protein, 1g fat, 200mg sodium (approx.)

- Total: 280 calories, 26g carbs, 18g protein, 12g fat, 340mg sodium (approx.)

Lunch:

- Turkey and Hummus Wrap (2 slices turkey, 2 tbsp hummus, lettuce, tomato, whole wheat wrap): 300 calories, 30g carbs, 22g protein, 10g fat, 600mg sodium (approx.)
- Orange (1 medium): 62 calories, 15g carbs, 1g protein, 0g fat, 0mg sodium

- Total: 362 calories, 45g carbs, 23g protein, 10g fat, 600mg sodium (approx.)

Dinner:
- Grilled Steak (4 oz): 250 calories, 0g carbs, 28g protein, 15g fat, 60mg sodium (approx.)
- Roasted Sweet Potatoes (1/2 cup): 90 calories, 20g carbs, 1g protein, 0g fat, 70mg sodium (approx.)
- Steamed Green Beans (1/2 cup): 20 calories, 4g carbs, 1g protein, 0g fat, 1mg sodium

- Total: 360 calories, 24g carbs, 30g protein, 15g fat, 131mg sodium (approx.)

Snack:
- Apple with Almond Butter (1 medium apple, 2 tbsp almond butter): 250 calories, 25g carbs, 4g protein, 16g fat, 0mg sodium

- Total: 250 calories, 25g carbs, 4g protein, 16g fat, 0mg sodium

Day 19
Breakfast:
- Whole Grain Pancakes with Berries (2 pancakes, 1/2 cup mixed berries): 260 calories, 52g carbs, 6g protein, 2g fat, 490mg sodium (approx.)

- Total: 260 calories, 52g carbs, 6g protein, 2g fat, 490mg sodium (approx.)

Lunch:
- Grilled Chicken Caesar Salad (4 oz grilled chicken breast, romaine lettuce, cherry tomatoes, Caesar dressing): 350 calories, 8g carbs, 40g protein, 18g fat, 700mg sodium (approx.)
- Whole Grain Breadstick: 100 calories, 20g carbs, 3g protein, 1g fat, 200mg sodium (approx.)

- Total: 450 calories, 28g carbs, 43g protein, 19g fat, 900mg sodium (approx.)

Dinner:
- Baked Tilapia (4 oz): 120 calories, 0g carbs, 23g protein, 3g fat, 55mg sodium (approx.)

- Quinoa (1/2 cup cooked): 111 calories, 19g carbs, 4g protein, 2g fat, 7mg sodium
- Steamed Broccoli (1/2 cup): 55 calories, 11g carbs, 4g protein, 1g fat, 30mg sodium (approx.)

- Total: 286 calories, 30g carbs, 31g protein, 6g fat, 92mg sodium (approx.)

Snack:
- Greek Yogurt with Honey (6 oz): 150 calories, 20g carbs, 11g protein, 0g fat, 70mg sodium (approx.)

- Total: 150 calories, 20g carbs, 11g protein, 0g fat, 70mg sodium (approx.)

Day 20
Breakfast:
- Greek Yogurt with Berries (6 oz Greek yogurt, 1/2 cup mixed berries): 150 calories, 20g carbs, 15g protein, 0g fat, 80mg sodium (approx.)

- Total: 150 calories, 20g carbs, 15g protein, 0g fat, 80mg sodium (approx.)

Lunch:

- Turkey and Avocado Wrap (2 slices turkey, 1/4 avocado, lettuce, tomato, whole wheat wrap): 300 calories, 30g carbs, 23g protein, 12g fat, 550mg sodium (approx.)
- Carrot Sticks (1 cup): 50 calories, 12g carbs, 1g protein, 0g fat, 70mg sodium (approx.)

- Total: 350 calories, 42g carbs, 24g protein, 12g fat, 620mg sodium (approx.)

Dinner:
- Grilled Salmon (4 oz): 220 calories, 0g carbs, 23g protein, 13g fat, 70mg sodium (approx.)
- Brown Rice (1/2 cup cooked): 108 calories, 22g carbs, 2g protein, 1g fat, 2mg sodium
- Steamed Broccoli (1/2 cup): 27 calories, 5g carbs, 2g protein, 0g fat, 30mg sodium (approx.)

- Total: 355 calories, 49g carbs, 27g protein, 14g fat, 102mg sodium (approx.)

Snack:
- Cottage Cheese (1/2 cup): 110 calories, 6g carbs, 14g protein, 4g fat, 400mg sodium (approx.)

- Total: 110 calories, 6g carbs, 14g protein, 4g fat, 400mg sodium (approx.)

Day 21
Breakfast:
- Oatmeal with Almond Milk (1/2 cup oats cooked in 1 cup almond milk): 180 calories, 30g carbs, 6g protein, 4g fat, 80mg sodium (approx.)
- Sliced Banana (1 medium): 105 calories, 27g carbs, 1g protein, 0g fat, 1mg sodium

- Total: 285 calories, 57g carbs, 7g protein, 4g fat, 81mg sodium (approx.)

Lunch:
- Tuna Salad (3 oz canned tuna, mixed greens, cherry tomatoes, cucumber, lemon juice): 150 calories, 3g carbs, 20g protein, 7g fat, 250mg sodium (approx.)
- Whole Grain Crackers (6 crackers): 120 calories, 20g carbs, 3g protein, 3g fat, 200mg sodium (approx.)

- Total: 270 calories, 23g carbs, 23g protein, 10g fat, 450mg sodium (approx.)

Dinner:

- Baked Chicken Breast (4 oz): 187 calories, 0g carbs, 35g protein, 4g fat, 85mg sodium (approx.)
- Quinoa (1/2 cup cooked): 111 calories, 19g carbs, 4g protein, 2g fat, 7mg sodium
- Steamed Asparagus (1/2 cup): 20 calories, 4g carbs, 2g protein, 0g fat, 0mg sodium

- Total: 318 calories, 23g carbs, 41g protein, 6g fat, 92mg sodium (approx.)

Snack:
- Apple Slices with Peanut Butter (1 medium apple, 2 tbsp peanut butter): 250 calories, 26g carbs, 5g protein, 16g fat, 0mg sodium

- Total: 250 calories, 26g carbs, 5g protein, 16g fat, 0mg sodium

Cooking Techniques to Reduce Sodium

Reducing sodium intake is a key dietary modification for managing Meniere's disease, as high levels of sodium can contribute to fluid retention and exacerbate symptoms. When preparing meals, it's essential to use cooking techniques that minimize the addition of sodium while enhancing flavor. Here are some cooking techniques to reduce sodium in your meals:

1. Flavorful Herbs and Spices: Instead of relying on salt for flavor, experiment with a variety of herbs and spices to enhance the taste of your dishes. Herbs like basil, thyme, oregano, and spices such as cumin, turmeric, and paprika can add depth and complexity to your meals without the need for extra salt.

2. Acidic Ingredients: Incorporate acidic ingredients like lemon juice, lime juice, vinegar, or tomatoes into your recipes. These ingredients can brighten flavors and provide a tangy contrast, reducing the need for added salt.

3. Homemade Seasonings: Create your own salt-free seasoning blends using a combination of dried herbs, spices, and aromatics. Store these blends in airtight containers for convenient use in various recipes.

4. Fresh Ingredients: Opt for fresh, whole ingredients whenever possible. Fresh vegetables, fruits, and meats are naturally lower in sodium compared to processed or pre-packaged foods.

5. Low-Sodium Broths and Stocks: Use low-sodium or sodium-free broths and stocks as a base for soups, stews, and sauces. These products are available in most grocery stores and can be used as a flavorful alternative to their high-sodium counterparts.

6. Rinsing and Soaking: If using canned beans or vegetables, rinse them thoroughly under running water to remove excess sodium. For dried beans, soak them overnight and rinse before cooking to reduce sodium content.

7. Limiting Salt During Cooking: When cooking, use minimal amounts of salt or omit it altogether. Instead, allow individuals to add salt to taste at the table, giving them more control over their sodium intake.

Chapter 4. Physical Therapy for

Meniere's Disease

Introduction to Vestibular Rehabilitation Therapy (VRT)

Vestibular Rehabilitation Therapy (VRT) is a specialized form of physical therapy designed to address balance and dizziness issues related to inner ear disorders, such as Meniere's disease. VRT focuses on exercises and techniques that promote central nervous system compensation for inner ear deficits, ultimately aiming to improve balance, reduce dizziness, and enhance overall vestibular function.

1. Goals of VRT:
   - VRT aims to achieve several goals, including:
     - Decreasing dizziness and vertigo symptoms
     - Improving balance and stability

- Enhancing gaze stability and visual focus during head movements
- Minimizing the impact of vestibular deficits on daily activities

2. Assessment and Customization in Vestibular Rehabilitation Therapy (VRT)

Initial Evaluation:
- The VRT process begins with an initial evaluation conducted by a trained physical therapist specializing in vestibular rehabilitation.
- During this evaluation, the therapist gathers detailed information about the individual's medical history, including the onset and progression of Meniere's disease symptoms, past treatments, and any other relevant health conditions.

Symptom Assessment:
- The therapist conducts a thorough assessment of the individual's specific symptoms related to Meniere's disease, including:
    - Frequency and duration of vertigo episodes
    - Severity of dizziness and imbalance
    - Presence and impact of associated symptoms such as nausea, vomiting, and visual disturbances

- Degree of functional impairment in daily activities due to vestibular symptoms

Functional Limitations:
- The therapist evaluates the individual's functional limitations related to balance and mobility, including:
- Ability to perform activities of daily living (e.g., walking, bending, reaching)
- Balance during static and dynamic tasks
- Risk of falls and fear of falling

Balance and Gait Assessment:
- Objective measures of balance and gait are often included in the assessment, using standardized tests and tools to quantify the individual's balance abilities.
- Tests may include assessments of standing balance, walking speed and stability, and dynamic balance tasks.

Visual and Vestibular Function Testing:
- The therapist may perform specific tests to assess the individual's visual and vestibular function, including:
- Visual acuity and tracking

- Vestibulo-ocular reflex (VOR) testing to evaluate the eyes' ability to stabilize vision during head movements
- Positional testing to assess for benign paroxysmal positional vertigo (BPPV), a common vestibular disorder that can coexist with Meniere's disease

Impact on Quality of Life:
- The assessment includes an evaluation of the impact of Meniere's disease on the individual's quality of life, including psychological and emotional factors.
- The therapist may use standardized questionnaires or interviews to assess aspects such as anxiety, depression, and overall well-being.

Goal Setting:
- Based on the assessment findings, the therapist collaborates with the individual to establish specific, measurable goals for VRT.
- Goals may include improving balance, reducing dizziness, increasing confidence in performing daily activities, and enhancing overall quality of life.

Customized Treatment Plan:
- Using the information gathered during the assessment, the therapist develops a customized

treatment plan tailored to the individual's needs, goals, and abilities.

- The treatment plan outlines the specific exercises, techniques, and strategies that will be employed during VRT to address the individual's symptoms and functional limitations.

3. Exercise Components:

- VRT exercises are designed to target specific vestibular and balance functions.

- Common exercises include:

- Habituation exercises: These involve repeated exposure to movements or positions that provoke dizziness, aiming to reduce sensitivity over time.

- Gaze stabilization exercises: These focus on improving visual focus and stability during head movements, helping to reduce symptoms like dizziness and disorientation.

- Balance training: These exercises aim to improve stability and proprioception, enhancing overall balance and reducing the risk of falls.

4. Progression and Monitoring:

- VRT is typically a progressive process, with exercises gradually increasing in complexity and difficulty as the individual's tolerance and abilities improve.

- Throughout the therapy process, the therapist monitors progress closely, adjusting the treatment plan as needed to ensure optimal outcomes.

5. Home Exercise Program:

- In addition to in-office sessions, individuals undergoing VRT are often prescribed a home exercise program to complement their therapy.

- Consistent practice of prescribed exercises at home is essential for maximizing the benefits of VRT.

Exercises for Balance Improvement

Vestibular rehabilitation therapy (VRT) is a specialized form of physical therapy that focuses on exercises and techniques to improve balance and reduce dizziness in individuals with vestibular disorders like Meniere's disease. These exercises are designed to promote central nervous system compensation for inner ear deficits and enhance the brain's ability to process balance information. Here are some common exercises used in VRT for balance improvement:

1. Gaze Stabilization Exercises:

- These exercises aim to improve visual stability during head movements, which can help reduce dizziness and improve balance.

- Example exercises include fixed-point staring, where you focus on a stationary object while moving your head side to side or up and down, and smooth pursuits, where you track a moving object with your eyes.

Step by step guide of Gaze Stabilization Exercises:

- Fixed-Point Staring:
- Pick a stationary object in your environment, such as a picture on the wall or a mark on the floor.
- Focus your gaze on the chosen point while gently moving your head from side to side, keeping your eyes fixed on the target.
- Repeat the movement several times, gradually increasing the speed of head movements as your ability improves.

- Vertical and Horizontal Head Movements:
- Choose a stationary object to focus on, such as a spot on the wall or a mark on the floor at eye level.
- Slowly move your head up and down while maintaining your gaze on the chosen target.

- Next, move your head from side to side while still keeping your eyes fixed on the target.

- Repeat these movements several times, ensuring smooth and controlled head movements.

- **Smooth Pursuits:**
- Hold an object, such as a pen or a finger, in front of you at arm's length.

- Slowly move the object horizontally in front of you, following its movement with your eyes while keeping your head still.

- Repeat the movement in the vertical direction, again following the object with your eyes only.

- Focus on maintaining smooth and steady eye movements throughout the exercise.

- **Rotational Head Movements:**
- Sit or stand in a comfortable position with a fixed gaze on a stationary object.

- Slowly rotate your head from side to side, keeping your eyes focused on the target.

- Gradually increase the speed and range of motion of your head movements while maintaining visual fixation.

- Return your head to the starting position and repeat the rotation several times.

- Target Tracking:

- Use a visual target, such as a moving object or a patterned background, placed at eye level.

- Track the movement of the target with your eyes while keeping your head still.

- Practice tracking the target in different directions, focusing on smooth and accurate eye movements.

- Increase the complexity of the tracking task by using faster or more unpredictable target movements.

2. Balance Training:

Balance exercises focus on improving stability and reducing the risk of falls.

Examples of Balance Training Exercises:

- Standing on One Leg:

- Stand on one leg while maintaining your balance.

- Hold the position for as long as you can, aiming for 30 seconds to 1 minute.

- Switch to the other leg and repeat the exercise.

- Walking in a Straight Line:

- Find a straight line on the ground, such as a crack in the sidewalk or a piece of tape on the floor.

- Walk along the line, placing one foot directly in front of the other, heel to toe.
- Focus on maintaining your balance and staying on the line without stepping off.

- Tandem Walking:
- Walk in a straight line, placing the heel of one foot directly in front of the toes of the other foot with each step.
- Continue this heel-to-toe pattern, maintaining a straight line and focusing on balance.

- Standing Up from a Seated Position:
- Sit in a chair with your feet flat on the floor and your hands on your lap.
- Without using your hands for support, stand up from the chair using only your leg muscles.
- Slowly sit back down, controlling the movement with your leg muscles.
- Repeat the process several times, focusing on smooth and controlled movements.

- Balancing on Unstable Surfaces:
- Use a balance pad, foam cushion, or wobble board to create an unstable surface.

- Stand on the unstable surface and focus on maintaining your balance.
- You can vary the difficulty by closing your eyes or performing other tasks while balancing.

- Heel-to-Toe Walk:
- Walk in a straight line, placing the heel of one foot directly in front of the toes of the other foot with each step.
- Maintain this heel-to-toe pattern, focusing on balance and coordination.
- You can perform this exercise along a straight line on the floor for added challenge.

3. Walking Exercises:
   Walking is a fundamental activity that can be used as a form of exercise to improve balance.

Examples of Walking Exercises for Balance Improvement:

- Walking on Uneven Surfaces:
- Find an area with uneven terrain, such as a grassy field or a hiking trail with natural obstacles.

- Walk carefully on the uneven surface, focusing on maintaining your balance and adapting to the changing terrain.
- Start with shorter distances and gradually increase the challenge as your balance improves.

- Navigating Obstacles:
- Set up a simple obstacle course using objects like cones, stepping stones, or small hurdles.
- Walk through the course, carefully stepping over or around each obstacle.
- Focus on maintaining a steady pace and adapting your movements to the obstacles in your path.

- Heel-to-Toe Walking:
- Walk in a straight line, placing the heel of one foot directly in front of the toes of the other foot with each step.
- Maintain this heel-to-toe pattern, focusing on balance and coordination.
- You can perform this exercise along a straight line on the floor or use a marked path for guidance.

- Backward Walking:
- Walk backward in a straight line, focusing on maintaining your balance and coordination.

- Start with short distances and gradually increase the distance as you become more comfortable with the movement.
- Use caution and ensure that the area is clear of obstacles when practicing backward walking.

- Sideways Walking:
- Walk sideways in a straight line, maintaining a steady pace and focusing on balance.
- You can vary the direction (left or right) to work both sides of the body evenly.
- Use caution and ensure that the area is clear of obstacles when practicing sideways walking.

4. Vestibular Habituation Exercises:
These exercises aim to reduce symptoms of dizziness and vertigo by gradually exposing the individual to movements or positions that provoke symptoms.

Examples of Vestibular Habituation Exercises:

- Head Movements:
- Slowly move your head in different directions, including up and down, side to side, and in circular motions.

- Start with slow, controlled movements and gradually increase the speed and range of motion.
- The goal is to habituate the vestibular system to these movements, reducing dizziness over time.

- **Positional Changes:**
- Practice transitioning between different positions, such as sitting to standing, lying down to sitting, or turning over in bed.
- These movements can provoke dizziness in individuals with vestibular disorders and are essential for habituation.

- **Balance Exercises with Head Movements:**
- Perform balance exercises, such as standing on one leg or on an unstable surface, while incorporating head movements.
- For example, you might try standing on one leg while slowly turning your head from side to side or up and down.

- **Gaze Stability Exercises:**
- Focus on a stationary object while moving your head in various directions.

- The goal is to maintain visual focus on the target despite head movements, which can help improve gaze stability and reduce dizziness.

- Visual Motion Exercises:
- Use visual stimuli that provoke dizziness, such as moving patterns or virtual reality simulations.
- Gradually increase exposure to these stimuli to desensitize the vestibular system and reduce symptoms over time.

- Walking and Turning:
- Practice walking in a straight line while turning your head from side to side.
- This exercise challenges the vestibular system by combining head movements with walking, helping to improve tolerance to these motions.

- Cervical Range of Motion Exercises:
- Perform exercises that focus on improving the range of motion in your neck.
- Gentle stretches and movements can help reduce muscle tension and improve flexibility, which can contribute to vestibular habituation.

5. Coordination and Agility Exercises:

These exercises focus on improving overall coordination and agility, which can contribute to better balance.

Examples of Coordination and Agility Exercises for Balance Improvement:

- Agility Ladder Drills:
- Set up an agility ladder on the ground (or create one using chalk or tape).
- Perform various footwork patterns, such as side shuffles, high knees, or quick steps, through the ladder.
- Focus on maintaining speed, accuracy, and coordination while moving through the ladder.

- Cone Drills:
- Place a series of cones or markers on the ground in a pattern or sequence.
- Perform drills that involve weaving in and out of the cones, circling around them, or changing direction quickly.
- These drills improve agility, balance, and the ability to change direction rapidly.

- Balance Board Exercises:

- Use a balance board or wobble board to perform exercises that challenge your balance.
- Stand on the board and practice maintaining your balance while performing tasks like reaching for objects or rotating your body.
- These exercises improve proprioception and overall stability.

- Reaction Drills:
- Use a partner or a coach to perform reaction drills that require quick responses to visual or auditory cues.
- For example, your partner might call out a direction, and you must quickly move in that direction.
- These drills improve reaction time and agility.

- Plyometric Exercises:
- Incorporate plyometric exercises like jumping, hopping, and bounding into your routine.
- Focus on explosive movements that require coordination and balance, such as jump squats or box jumps.
- These exercises improve lower body power and agility.

- Obstacle Courses:

- Set up an obstacle course with various challenges like hurdles, cones, and balance beams.
- Navigate through the course, focusing on maintaining balance and coordination while overcoming obstacles.
- Obstacle courses improve agility, spatial awareness, and coordination.

- Circuit Training:
- Design a circuit that includes a variety of exercises targeting different muscle groups and movement patterns.
- Perform each exercise in the circuit for a set amount of time or repetitions before moving to the next.
- Circuit training improves overall fitness, including coordination, agility, and balance.

6. Tai Chi and Yoga:
   Tai Chi and yoga are mind-body exercises that emphasize balance, flexibility, and controlled movements.
   These practices can complement traditional VRT exercises and provide additional benefits for balance improvement and overall well-being.

Tai Chi Exercises:

1. "Cloud Hands" (Yun Shou):
   - Start in a relaxed standing position with your feet shoulder-width apart and your knees slightly bent.
   - Begin by shifting your weight to your right leg and turning your torso to the right, allowing your arms to follow in a circular motion.
   - As you shift your weight to your left leg, continue the circular motion of your arms to the left.
   - Repeat this flowing motion, coordinating the movement of your arms with the shifting of your weight from one leg to the other.
   - Focus on maintaining a relaxed and flowing rhythm throughout the exercise.

2. "Repulse Monkey" (Dao Nian Hou):
   - Begin in a standing position with your feet shoulder-width apart and your knees slightly bent.
   - Shift your weight to your right leg and step back with your left foot, keeping your toes pointed slightly outward.
   - As you step back, turn your torso to the left and extend your arms in front of you, palms facing outward.

- Shift your weight back to your left leg, bringing your right foot back to the starting position.

- Repeat this sequence, alternating sides with each repetition.

- Focus on maintaining a smooth and controlled movement, coordinating the stepping and arm movements.

3. "Grasp the Sparrow's Tail" (Lan Que Wei):

- Begin in a standing position with your feet shoulder-width apart and your knees slightly bent.

- Start with your arms relaxed at your sides.

- Shift your weight to your right leg and step back with your left foot, keeping your toes pointed slightly outward.

- As you step back, turn your torso to the left and extend your arms in front of you, palms facing outward.

- Shift your weight back to your left leg, bringing your right foot back to the starting position.

- Repeat this sequence, alternating sides with each repetition.

- Focus on maintaining a smooth and controlled movement, coordinating the stepping and arm movements.

Yoga Exercises:

1. Tree Pose (Vrikshasana):
  - Begin in a standing position with your feet together and your arms at your sides.
  - Shift your weight onto your left foot and lift your right foot off the ground.
  - Place the sole of your right foot on the inner left thigh or calf, avoiding the knee joint.
  - Press your foot into your leg and your leg into your foot to create a stable base.
  - Bring your palms together in front of your chest in a prayer position, or raise your arms overhead.
  - Hold the pose for 30 seconds to 1 minute, then switch sides.

2. Warrior III Pose (Virabhadrasana III):
  - Begin in a standing position with your feet hip-width apart and your arms at your sides.
  - Shift your weight onto your left foot and lift your right foot off the ground.
  - Hinge forward at the hips, extending your right leg behind you and reaching your arms forward.
  - Keep your hips and shoulders square to the ground, and your body forming a straight line from head to heel.

- Hold the pose for 30 seconds to 1 minute, then switch sides.

3. Half Moon Pose (Ardha Chandrasana):
   - Begin in a standing position with your feet together and your arms at your sides.
   - Step your left foot back about 3-4 feet and turn your left foot out about 45 degrees.
   - Extend your arms out to the sides at shoulder height.
   - Shift your weight onto your right foot and lift your left leg off the ground.
   - Rotate your torso to the left and bring your left arm down to the floor, either inside or outside of your right foot.
   - Extend your right arm toward the ceiling, creating a "half moon" shape with your body.
   - Hold the pose for 30 seconds to 1 minute, then switch sides.

Gaze Stabilization Exercises

1. Fixed Gaze Technique:
   - Find a stationary object to focus on, such as a spot on the wall or a small object held at eye level.

- Stand or sit in a comfortable position with your head facing forward and your eyes on the target.
- Slowly move your head from side to side, keeping your eyes fixed on the target.
- Repeat the head movements several times, gradually increasing the speed and range of motion.
- If you experience dizziness or discomfort, slow down or stop the movements and rest before continuing.

2. Smooth Pursuit Technique:
- Choose a visual target, such as a finger or a small object, and hold it at arm's length.
- Keep your head still and focus on the target with your eyes.
- Move the target smoothly in a horizontal or vertical path while tracking it with your eyes.
- Follow the target's movements as accurately as possible, maintaining a steady gaze.
- Repeat the tracking movements in different directions, gradually increasing the speed and complexity of the movements.

3. Vestibulo-Ocular Reflex (VOR) Exercises:
- Sit in a chair with your eyes focused on a distant object.

- Turn your head to the right and then back to the center while keeping your eyes fixed on the target.
- Repeat the head turns to the left and back to the center.
- Increase the speed of the head turns gradually, maintaining focus on the target throughout the movements.
- You can also perform these exercises with whole-body movements, such as turning your entire body to look over your shoulder while keeping your eyes on a fixed point.

4. Adaptation Exercises:
- These exercises are typically performed under the guidance of a physical therapist.
- They may involve specific movements or activities designed to induce controlled dizziness or challenge your balance.
- Your therapist will gradually increase the intensity and duration of these exercises as your tolerance improves.

5. Progressive Challenges:
- As you become more proficient in the basic gaze stabilization exercises, your therapist may introduce more challenging variations.

- These may include performing the exercises on unstable surfaces (like foam pads or balance boards) or in environments with increased sensory input (such as busy visual environments).

Always consult with a qualified physical therapist before starting any new exercise program, especially if you have a medical condition like Meniere's disease. They can provide personalized guidance and ensure that the exercises are safe and appropriate for your specific needs.

Chapter 5. Stress Management

Techniques

Understanding the Link Between Stress and Meniere's Symptoms

Stress can have a significant impact on the symptoms of Meniere's disease, often exacerbating the frequency and severity of vertigo episodes, tinnitus, and other associated symptoms. While stress itself may not directly cause Meniere's disease, it can act as a trigger or amplifier for existing symptoms. Understanding the link between stress and Meniere's symptoms is essential for developing effective stress management strategies. Here's how stress can influence Meniere's disease:

1. Effects on the Vestibular System: Stress can affect the function of the vestibular system, which is responsible for balance and spatial orientation.

Increased stress levels may lead to changes in the vestibular system's sensitivity, making individuals more susceptible to vertigo attacks and feelings of imbalance.

2. Impact on Blood Flow: Stress can affect blood flow in the inner ear, potentially disrupting the delicate balance of fluids and pressure that is crucial for normal inner ear function. This disruption may contribute to symptoms such as ear fullness and tinnitus.

3. Muscle Tension and Posture: Stress can cause muscle tension, particularly in the neck and shoulders, which can affect posture and contribute to neck-related issues that may exacerbate Meniere's symptoms. Poor posture can also affect blood flow and nerve function, potentially impacting symptoms.

4. Emotional Well-being: The emotional toll of living with a chronic condition like Meniere's disease can be significant. Stress, anxiety, and depression are common among individuals with Meniere's, and these emotional states can exacerbate symptoms and reduce overall quality of life.

5. Coping Strategies: Developing effective coping strategies for managing stress is crucial for individuals with Meniere's disease. By learning how to reduce stress levels and cope with stressors effectively, individuals can potentially reduce the impact of stress on their symptoms.

6. Stress Triggers: Identifying specific stressors that can trigger or worsen Meniere's symptoms is important for managing stress. Common stressors may include work-related pressures, family issues, financial concerns, or health-related worries.

7. The Role of Relaxation: Engaging in relaxation techniques such as deep breathing, progressive muscle relaxation, meditation, or yoga can help reduce stress levels and promote a sense of calm. These techniques can be particularly beneficial during times of increased stress or when symptoms are exacerbated.

Relaxation Techniques: Meditation and Breathing Exercises

Stress management is an essential aspect of managing Meniere's disease, as stress can exacerbate symptoms and impact overall well-being. Incorporating relaxation techniques into daily life can help individuals with Meniere's reduce stress levels and improve their ability to cope with the challenges of the condition. Two effective relaxation techniques are meditation and breathing exercises:

1. Meditation:
   - Meditation is a practice that involves focusing the mind and eliminating distractions to achieve a state of relaxation and mental clarity.
   - Guided meditation, mindfulness meditation, and mantra meditation are popular techniques that can be practiced individually or with the help of audio guides or apps.
   - Benefits of meditation for individuals with Meniere's disease may include reduced stress levels, improved mental focus, and better emotional regulation.

Techniques:

Here's a step-by-step guide for practicing meditation techniques, including guided meditation, mindfulness meditation, and mantra meditation:

- Guided Meditation:

  - Find a quiet and comfortable place where you can sit or lie down without distractions.
  - Close your eyes and take a few deep breaths to relax your body and mind.
  - Start the guided meditation recording or app of your choice.
  - Follow the instructions of the guide, which may involve visualizations, breathing exercises, or body scans.
  - Focus on the guide's voice and the instructions, allowing yourself to let go of any thoughts or distractions.
  - Continue to follow the guide's instructions until the meditation session is complete.
  - Take a few moments to rest and notice how you feel before returning to your usual activities.

- Mindfulness Meditation:

  - Find a comfortable seated position with your back straight but relaxed.
  - Close your eyes or gaze softly at a spot in front of you.
  - Begin by bringing your attention to your breath, noticing the sensation of the breath as it enters and leaves your body.

- As thoughts, sensations, or emotions arise, acknowledge them without judgment and gently bring your focus back to your breath.
- Continue to observe your breath, returning to it whenever your mind wanders.
- Practice this for a predetermined amount of time, such as 5 or 10 minutes, gradually increasing the duration as you become more comfortable with the practice.
- When you're ready, slowly open your eyes and take a moment to transition back to your surroundings.

- Mantra Meditation:
- Choose a word, phrase, or sound (mantra) that resonates with you and has positive associations.
- Find a comfortable seated position with your back straight but relaxed.
- Close your eyes and take a few deep breaths to center yourself.
- Begin silently repeating your chosen mantra with each breath, focusing on the sound or feeling of the mantra.
- If your mind wanders, gently bring your focus back to the mantra without judgment.
- Continue to repeat the mantra for a predetermined amount of time, such as 5 or 10 minutes.

- When you're ready, slowly release the mantra and take a few moments to rest before returning to your usual activities.

2. Breathing Exercises:

- Breathing exercises, also known as deep breathing or diaphragmatic breathing, can help calm the mind and body by promoting relaxation and reducing the body's stress response.

- To practice deep breathing, individuals should find a comfortable position and focus on taking slow, deep breaths in through the nose, filling the abdomen with air, and then exhaling slowly through the mouth.

- Deep breathing can be practiced anywhere and anytime, making it a convenient and accessible stress management technique.

Technique:

- Find a Comfortable Position:
  - Sit or lie down in a comfortable position, with your back straight but relaxed. You can also practice deep breathing while standing if that's more comfortable for you.

- Relax Your Body:
    - Close your eyes if you're comfortable doing so, and take a few moments to relax your body. Release any tension in your muscles, starting from your head and working down to your toes.

- Focus on Your Breath:
    - Begin to pay attention to your breath without trying to control it. Notice the natural rhythm of your breathing, the rise and fall of your chest or abdomen with each breath.

- Inhale Slowly Through Your Nose:
    - Take a slow, deep breath in through your nose, allowing your abdomen to expand as you fill your lungs with air. Try to inhale for a count of 4 or 5 seconds, or whatever feels comfortable for you.

- Exhale Slowly Through Your Mouth:
    - Exhale slowly and completely through your mouth, allowing your abdomen to contract as you release the air from your lungs. Try to exhale for a count of 4 or 5

seconds, or whatever feels comfortable for you.

- Repeat:
  - Continue this slow, deep breathing pattern, focusing on the sensation of your breath as it enters and leaves your body. Inhale deeply, exhale completely, and pause briefly before the next breath.

- Counting Your Breaths:
  - If it helps you focus, you can count your breaths. For example, count silently to yourself as you inhale (1, 2, 3, 4), hold your breath for a moment, and then count as you exhale (1, 2, 3, 4).

- Practice for Several Minutes:
  - Practice deep breathing for several minutes, gradually increasing the duration as you become more comfortable with the technique. Aim for 5 to 10 minutes initially, and you can extend the duration as you feel more at ease.

- Transition Back to Normal Breathing:
    - When you're ready to finish, take a few normal breaths and gradually return to your regular breathing pattern. Notice how you feel after practicing deep breathing.

- Practice Regularly:
    - To experience the benefits of deep breathing, practice this technique regularly. You can incorporate deep breathing into your daily routine, such as before bedtime or during moments of stress or anxiety.

3. Incorporating Relaxation Techniques Into Daily Life:

- Setting aside dedicated time for meditation or breathing exercises each day can be beneficial for managing stress and promoting relaxation.

- Integrating these techniques into daily routines, such as practicing deep breathing before bedtime or meditating during a break at work, can help make them a regular part of one's lifestyle.

- Experimenting with different types of meditation and breathing exercises to find what works best for individual preferences and needs is encouraged.

4. Consistency and Persistence:

   - Like any skill, mastering relaxation techniques requires practice and patience.

   - Consistent practice of meditation and breathing exercises can lead to long-term benefits in managing stress and improving overall well-being.

Chapter 6. Integrative

Approaches

Acupuncture and Acupressure for Symptom Management

Acupuncture and acupressure are traditional Chinese medicine techniques that have been used for centuries to manage various health conditions, including symptoms associated with Meniere's disease. While research on their specific effects on Meniere's disease is still limited, some individuals with Meniere's have reported finding relief from certain symptoms through these techniques. Here's how acupuncture and acupressure may be used for symptom management in Meniere's disease:

1. Acupuncture: Acupuncture involves the insertion of thin needles into specific points on the body to stimulate energy flow and promote healing. In the

context of Meniere's disease, acupuncture may be used to target symptoms such as vertigo, tinnitus, and nausea. Some studies suggest that acupuncture may help improve blood flow to the inner ear and regulate the body's response to stress, potentially reducing the frequency and severity of vertigo attacks.

2. Acupressure: Acupressure is a technique that involves applying pressure to specific points on the body using the fingers, thumbs, or specialized devices. Like acupuncture, acupressure aims to stimulate the body's natural healing processes. Acupressure points that may be targeted for Meniere's disease include those believed to be associated with the ear, balance, and stress regulation. By applying pressure to these points, individuals may experience relief from symptoms such as vertigo and anxiety.

Potential Benefits:
While the scientific evidence supporting the use of acupuncture and acupressure for Meniere's disease is still emerging, some individuals report finding these techniques helpful in managing their symptoms. Acupuncture and acupressure are generally considered safe when performed by trained

practitioners, and they may offer a non-invasive and drug-free option for symptom management.

Considerations:
It's essential for individuals considering acupuncture or acupressure for Meniere's disease to work with a qualified practitioner who has experience in treating this condition. Additionally, these techniques should be used as complementary approaches alongside conventional medical treatment, rather than as a replacement for it. It's important to consult with a healthcare provider before starting any new treatment, especially if you have a pre-existing medical condition or are taking medications.

Personalized Approach:
As with any treatment for Meniere's disease, the effectiveness of acupuncture and acupressure can vary from person to person. Some individuals may find these techniques beneficial as part of a comprehensive treatment plan, while others may not experience significant relief. It's essential to approach integrative approaches like acupuncture and acupressure with an open mind and a willingness to explore what works best for your individual needs.

Herbal Remedies and Supplements: What to Consider

Many individuals with Meniere's disease explore complementary and alternative medicine (CAM) approaches, including herbal remedies and supplements, to manage their symptoms. While some herbs and supplements may offer potential benefits, it's essential to approach their use with caution and under the guidance of a healthcare provider. Here are some considerations when considering herbal remedies and supplements for Meniere's disease:

1. Consultation with a Healthcare Provider: Before starting any herbal remedy or supplement, it's crucial to consult with a healthcare provider, especially if you are taking medications or have underlying health conditions. Some herbs and supplements can interact with medications or may not be safe for certain individuals.

2. Research and Evidence: Look for herbs and supplements that have been studied for their potential benefits in managing Meniere's disease. While some herbs may have traditional use in managing certain symptoms, it's important to seek

out scientific evidence to support their efficacy and safety.

3. Quality and Safety: Choose products from reputable manufacturers that adhere to quality and safety standards. Look for third-party certifications, such as Good Manufacturing Practice (GMP) or NSF International, which ensure that the product has been tested for purity and potency.

4. Commonly Studied Herbs and Supplements: Some herbs and supplements that have been studied in the context of Meniere's disease include:
   - Ginkgo biloba: Thought to improve blood flow to the inner ear, potentially reducing symptoms like vertigo and tinnitus.
   - Vitamin B6 (pyridoxine): Some studies suggest that vitamin B6 supplementation may help reduce the frequency and severity of vertigo attacks.
   - Magnesium: Magnesium deficiency has been linked to certain vestibular disorders, and supplementation may help alleviate symptoms.

5. Potential Risks and Side Effects: Be aware of potential risks and side effects associated with herbs and supplements. For example, ginkgo biloba may

increase the risk of bleeding, especially in individuals taking blood-thinning medications.

6. Individualized Approach: Everyone responds differently to herbs and supplements, so it's essential to approach their use on an individualized basis. Keep track of any changes in symptoms or side effects when starting a new herbal remedy or supplement.

7. Integration with Conventional Treatment: Herbal remedies and supplements should not replace conventional medical treatment for Meniere's disease. They should be viewed as complementary to other treatment strategies, and their use should be discussed with a healthcare provider as part of a comprehensive management plan.